A Study Guide

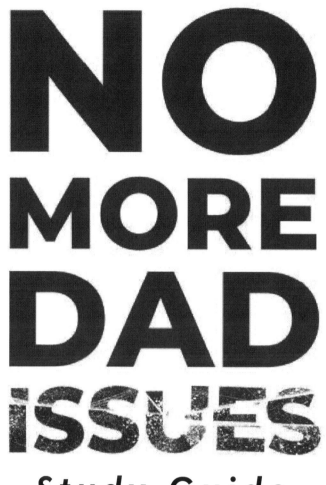

NO MORE DAD ISSUES

Study Guide

DAVE NOVAK

Copyright © 2023 By David Novak. All rights reserved.

No part of this work may be reproduced, stored in a retrieval system, or transmitted in any form by any means, electronic, mechanical, photocopying, recording, or otherwise, without the written permission of the author. The use of short quotes is permitted and encouraged for the use of a person or group study. For rights and permissions, contact the author using the information below.

Confidentiality Statement: Those with their real names in the book have permitted the author to appear in print. In order to protect the confidentiality of other individuals, some names have been changed or intentionally omitted.

Dave Novak Ministries
5050 Laguna Blvd. Unit 112 #770 Elk Grove, California
Email: dave@davenovakministries.com Website: Davenovakministrties.com

Book cover by Nskvsky. Edited by Chrissa Unterberger and Brianna Reisenwitz

Italics or bold lettering are used to indicate emphasis, narration, or thoughts of the author.

Scripture

All scripture quotations, unless otherwise indicated, are taken from the Holy Bible, New International Version (NIV). Copyright © 1973, 1978, 1984, 2011 by Biblica, Inc. Used by permission of Zondervan. Other Bible versions used include the following, and are indicated in the text. New American Standard Bible® (NAS), Copyright © 1960, 1971, 1977, 1995, 2020 by The Lockman Foundation. Used by permission. J.B. Phillips New Testament (PHILLIPS), Copyright© 1962, by HarperCollins. New Living Translation (NLT), Copyright © 1996, 2004, 2015 by Tyndale House Foundation. New Century Version (NCV), Copyright © 2005 by Thomas Nelson. Used by permission. New King James Version (NKJV), Copyright © 1982 by Thomas Nelson. Amplified Bible, Classic Edition (AMPC), Copyright © 1954, 1958, 1962, 1964, 1965, 1987 by TheLockman Foundation. The Message (MSG), Copyright 1993, 1994, 1995, 1996, 2000, 2001, 2002. Used by permission of NavPress Publishing Group. English Standard Version (ESV), Copyright © 2001 by Crossway Bibles. The Living Bible (TLB), Copyright © 1971 by Tyndale House.

DEDICATION

To Leah and Titus, you inspire me to be the best dad I can be. You're the joys of my life. I'm proud to be your dad.

TABLE OF CONTENTS

A Note from Pastor Dave 9

Getting Started (How to Use) 11

Session #1: Discovering Who Really Has the Issue 13

Session #2: Facing Hurts from a Flawed Hero (Part 1) 26

Session #3: Facing Hurts from a Flawed Hero (Part 2) 38

Session #4: Seeing Through the Eyes of Mercy 51

Session #5: Quitting the Blame Game 65

Session #6: Planning Freedom for a Greater Future 78

In Closing from Pastor Dave 90

About the Author 91

A NOTE FROM PASTOR DAVE

You are about to embark on one of the most healing journeys you have ever been on in your life! The fact you have spent money on the "No More Dad Issues" book along with this study guide and are willing to spend lots of time going through it says you are ready. I love hearing the testimonies from individuals who have found freedom due to reading the book. *You, too,* will have a great testimony as you see this guide to the end.

When I initially wrote "No More Dad Issues," I didn't plan on writing anything else. But as I continued to hear how people have been impacted, I felt an urgency birthed in my spirit, saying, *"We've gotta do more!"*

This book is meant to take you in-depth into your hurts and frustrations with your dad, identify them, learn how they're affecting your life, and then make corrections to be liberated from this burden. The wounds and scars from your father may not immediately disappear, but I am confident that your view of your relationship with your dad and your relationships with others will improve. You will be a stronger and healthier version of yourself.

As you are confronted with hard questions in each session, they are part of the healing process. Like any physical wound, initial care from a doctor may not be pleasant, but it helps prevent the injury from getting worse. Then, it's about maintaining the instructions and prescriptions the doctor gives to recover.

I'm blessed by your courage and energy to move forward. I believe in God's gracious touch on your future.

GETTING STARTED (HOW TO USE)

As you'll discover in this study, healing, and freedom are attainable. This is not directed to a certain demographic. It can be used by women, men, and even teenagers.

This is not to be a burden like homework. This book is meant to be a tool to enable individuals to process the past and lean on what it will take to have new, fresh perspectives. But the truth is, the more you put into it, the more you will get out of it. In each section, there are corresponding chapters referred to in "No More Dad Issues" that will enrich your experience if you include them. This can also be used to follow up on reading you did in the past.

This is a book study and a Bible study. *"For the word of God is living and active. Sharper than any double-edged sword, it penetrates even to dividing soul and spirit, joints and marrow; it judges the thoughts and attitudes of the heart"* (Hebrews 4:12). Without God's Living Word, it's almost impossible to have change and effect growth. In each section, relevant passages are provided for you to personalize and receive principles directly from the Bible. There will be truths for you to turn to for future guidance in your area of hurt.

The guide can be used in a variety of formats. It can be used as a personal study, a study with a couple close friends, or in a larger small group ministry.

Ask the Holy Spirit to reveal areas needing healing and learn how your Heavenly Father wants to bring healing.

This is going to be amazing. Let the great journey begin!

——— SESSION #1 ———

DISCOVERING WHO REALLY HAS THE ISSUE

> "An overwhelming number of people have experienced a "love deficit" from their father. Because of this deficit, there are wounded areas in your soul"
>
> **NO MORE DAD ISSUES, PAGE XIV**

UNCOVERING ISSUES

It's amazing what you find when you move furniture placed in the same areas for years. You can now see the items you've looked for under the couch. Maybe traces of food remnants. Dust and traces of dirt. Unfortunately, there are pieces of food leaving that smell you could never discover where it was coming from. If you never look, you'll never remedy the mess, and it may take some extra effort to make everything right.

When considering dad issues, they're not things we look forward to uncovering. We know these issues come with wounds or frustrations.

Who wants to relive wounds received from their father? Who wants to remember situations that injured your heart? These areas are often avoided, denied, or ignored because the pain is too great. So, we unknowingly carry the emotions and burdens we haven't been able to heal from and even be released from.

As we continually overlook the past and the damage dad issues have created for us, we look for an alternative target for relief. We build up resentment and bitterness towards the person who initiated the pain. When we dismiss the issues we have never dealt with, they develop toxic and dysfunctional outcomes in several areas of our lives.

These issues, when left uncovered, breed greater problems for us; they are too heavy for you to bear.

- As you reflect on your relationship with your dad, have you avoided "digging in" to any pain? Why?

- How long have you resisted exploring the negative effects that have come from your dad's actions towards you? What has influenced the resistance?

- Do you believe you have issues with your dad's involvement, or lack thereof, in your life? Explain.

> "Consider your own relationship with your dad. How is your heart when you think about the condition of love from or toward your dad?
>
> Maybe your dad neglected you and your emotional needs. Is there conflict, and you can't stand to be near him? Was he an absentee father and didn't go out of his way to be a support to you? Did addictions and substance abuse steal him away from you? Maybe you experienced some sort of abuse from another person, and he didn't do anything to stand up for you. Or maybe you had a father who put his career in front of you. Perhaps you were a pastor's kid, like me, and saw your father tirelessly going out of his way to care for others at your expense. Or perhaps you have never met your dad because he decided to live life without you. It's possible you lost your father at a young age and decided to deal with the pain on your own.
>
> There's an endless number of possible ways we can feel pain related to, or caused by, our fathers. These are heavy burdens that can lead us to feel desperate for change, or worse, hopeless."
>
> **NO MORE DAD ISSUES, PAGE 13**

- Do any of these occurrences from this excerpt resonate with you or initiate a memory in your relationship with your dad? Describe.

- Describe the emotions you have as you recall these experiences. (sadness, hurt, anger, etc.)

This scripture communicates what we haven't been released from will continually overpower our desires and ambitions. This includes your desire to live healthy and free.

2 Peter 2:19 says, "*A man is a slave to whatever has mastered him.*"

- List your dad's words and/or actions that have injured you over the years.

- The unresolved issues with our dads become the owners of many areas in our lives if left unaddressed. As you reflect, can you see the wounds have mastered you? Share an experience that reveals how they have mastered you.

- How do you believe issues and troubles with your dad have weighed you down? (In family relationships, workplaces, friendships, etc.)

CONFRONTING ISSUES

Throughout the book, Dave reveals his frustrations and ill feelings towards his dad. The underlying tension came from the changes needing to take place, but his dad didn't initiate restoration. Thus, Dave never realized these necessary changes, so his bitterness and hopelessness multiplied over time because he didn't have the ability to change his dad.

DAVE NOVAK

Since Dave could not bring change, he unknowingly resorted to blaming his dad for not making things right. He couldn't let his father "off the hook" for not making things right. Dave would find himself defeated because his brokenness would never find relief. For him, there was no way out.

- As you reflect, have you naturally blamed your dad for the brokenness you feel? In what ways?

- As Dave did, have you felt helpless and hopeless in your pursuit of healing and freedom? Explain.

In the following excerpt from No More Dad Issues, Dave eventually discovers he has been believing a lie. This lie had kept him from wholeness

> "This lie kept me bound for years, captive by my own heartbreak and anger. I'm convinced this one lie creates heavy burdens for numerous others who have similar issues. Until we're able to stare this lie in the face and confront reality in our minds, we will not be able to find freedom from dad issues. The lie so many of us believe is that the issue is HIS issue, and if Dad would simply take responsibility for HIS issue, then we'd overcome what has been defeating us. The logic of the lie tells us that if Dad created the issue, he should fix it. To undo the lie, I had to learn a hard truth: the issues in the relationship with my dad were now MY issues."
>
> **NO MORE DAD ISSUES, PAGE 15**

- Have you believed the "Big Lie"? Why?

- In this excerpt, we realize that our dads are owners of the offenses, but we are owners of the issues. Do you agree or disagree with this statement? Why?

- Have you ever considered your "issues" are not your dad's but yours? How does that impact your perspective moving forward?

- How does it feel to know the only way for you to be free from dad issues is for you to do something about them?

Robert Anthony, a professor at Harvard Business School, once stated: *"When you blame others, you give up your power to change."*

- If this statement holds true, are you willing to stop blaming for the possibility of change in you?

- What are ways you've been blaming and now need to correct?

- Are you willing to work on your brokenness and find healing even if your dad never changes?

RESOLVING ISSUES

Mending our issues can no longer be placed on the person who has been causing the offenses if we want to heal. We can try to persuade them to understand their need to be responsible for our hurts and, more likely, remain empty. Our new source of healing and restoration in our hearts is found in Christ. He alone can trade his healing for our wounds. In these teaching passages, Jesus explains how we can find rest in our souls by turning to him.

> *Come to Me, all you who labor and are heavy-laden and overburdened, and I will cause you to rest. [I will ease and relieve and refresh your souls.] Take My yoke upon you and learn of Me,*

> *for I am gentle (meek) and humble (lowly) in heart, and you will find rest (relief and ease and refreshment and recreation and blessed quiet) for your souls. For my yoke is wholesome (useful, good—not harsh, hard, sharp, or pressing, but comfortable, gracious, and pleasant), and my burden is light and easy to bear.*
>
> **MATTHEW 11:28-30 (AMP)**

- Do you believe, due to your relationship with your dad, you have lived an "overburdened" life to some degree? In what ways?

- Describe how you feel when Jesus promises to give us rest and relief from our burdens.

- Are you ready to unload your heartache and give it to Christ? What will make that difficult?

OVERCOMING ISSUES

Vision is a motivator. We are more likely to pursue change when we envision what could be and should be. If you don't envision being debt-free, you won't cut back on spending. If you don't envision a better marriage, you won't work on your communication skills. If you don't envision earning your Masters, you probably won't push through the difficult study times to get a passing grade.

On the flip side, when we don't have a vision, our life is aimless and unproductive; we easily give up and can even become dysfunctional.

If you want restoration in your soul, you'll need to see what it would be like and visualize the steps you must take to be whole.

> "The only way there is hope on the horizon for healing and freedom is to get a new vision. It's a new vision only God can provide. Proverbs 29:18 reads, "Where there is no vision, the people cast off restraint." If we can't have a transformed vision in our hearts, it will lead us to run wild and maintain a life of hurt and destruction, which will spread like cancer."
>
> **NO MORE DAD ISSUES, PAGE 15**

- Do you believe your life will continue down a hurtful path if you don't make changes? How?

- List five ways your life would be better if you could break free from your dad's issues.

- What needs to change for you to heal and break free from your dad's issues?

TRANSFORMING ISSUES

1 Peter 5:7 (TLB) Let him (God) have all your worries and cares, for he is always thinking about you and watching everything that concerns you.

- The phrase, "he is always thinking about you," reveals how much God values you. Have you always felt your life had value?

- If God cares about all your worries and suffering, what does that say about his love for you?

- How does this scripture encourage and comfort you as you begin this new journey towards healing and freedom?

―――― **SESSION #2** ――――

FACING HURTS FROM A FLAWED HERO (PART 1)

> "I wanted my dad to be a hero in the home. That's all I ever wanted my dad to be."
>
> **NO MORE DAD ISSUES, PAGE 51**

Book Reading: Part II 6-8

Considering Reading 2 Samuel 13:1-29 in your Bible

UNCOVERING ISSUES

King David was the hero of a nation in so many ways. He had conquered numerous opposing nations who threatened Israel. He conquered the mighty Philistine champion Goliath, winning one of the greatest wars ever. He was the underdog who became the Cinderella story. David's great exploits go on and on. Hero was too much of a basic and vague term. But when you enter David's home, his role is anything but heroic.

So much dysfunction filled David's home. Due to the often toxic environment, David lacks high admiration in that arena. Since there were defeats in his fathering, hurt didn't follow far behind, leaving wounds and scars in the hearts of his children.

What do you do when the hero you admire is also the source of your hurts? Where do you turn for healing and freedom? This pain is still alive and pervasive today. We naturally grow up wanting a hero.

Proverbs 17:6 (ESV) states, *"The glory of children is their fathers."* This passage reinforces how children view their fathers as heroes. It's part of our divine makeup.

- In your own words, how would you describe the characteristics of a heroic dad?

- Do you think your dad knew he had hurt you? How was that reflected?

- How have you handled the hurts from your dad?

In the book, Dave reveals in practical and relevant ways that he was not fulfilling his role as a desired hero.

> "After a rape and intense hate morphed in Absalom's heart, nothing happened for two years. As such, Absalom decided to take things into his own hands. David didn't discipline Amnon for his crime. Tamar received no justice for the assault against her. The father in the home brought neither leadership nor nurturing to his children. Instead, he neglected his kids and left them to do as they saw fit.
>
> What's interesting is that prior to "Two years later," it reads, "When David heard all this, he was furious." That means David knew all about the crime. It hurt his heart and made him grieved and angry. But David didn't do anything about the dysfunction in his home. Failure to act is a failure to lead."
>
> **NO MORE DAD ISSUES, PAGE 61**

- What might the feelings of David's children be in response to his fathering?

- Did you ever feel abandoned or neglected by your dad? If so, in what ways?

> For so many generations today, wounds are pervasive in a variety of ways. You may even identify with the circumstances Dave describes in this excerpt that contribute to your development of dad issues.
>
> "What about dads who chose to never be around and take responsibility? Those who may be described in some circles as, only "baby daddies," and "deadbeat dads." They leave when a child is young to run wild. They don't pay child support, chase other relationships, use drugs, or abuse other substances.
>
> Careers have robbed kids of their dads. Men can be so ambitious that they will even risk losing their kids. They may have climbed the ladder of success only to find out later it was leaning against the wrong wall."
>
> **NO MORE DAD ISSUES PAGE 68**

- What types of painful emotions can grow from circumstances with dads such as these?

- In the past, did you ever possess the "you don't care, and neither do I" mentality? Why?

Many times, when our dads don't show up, it's not only physically present but emotionally distant or even wounds inflicted. Because of this, bitterness develops.

Colossians 3:21 clearly describes how this can come about: *"Fathers, do not provoke or irritate or fret your children [do not be hard on them or harass them], lest they become discouraged and sullen and morose and feel inferior and frustrated. [Do not break their spirit.]"*

- Do you believe your dad knew he was doing this to your spirit or even cared? How could he have changed it?

- Can you attribute careless decisions and behaviors to the way your dad treated you? What are some of those things?

> "Bitterness is probably the highest populated prison ever known to man. It doesn't even need security because the inmates will hold themselves there for a life sentence by their own choice. They never plan to break out.'
> **NO MORE DAD ISSUES, PAGE 75**

- Has bitterness been a prison for you? Describe how.

- If you have bitterness stored up, are you willing to release it? Why or why not?

CONFRONTING ISSUES

> In the story of David and his family, his son Absalom didn't address his ill feelings and pain toward his dad to his demise.
>
> Physical wounds and scars come in all shapes and sizes. Emotional wounds and scars aren't very different; they just can't be seen. With all injuries, if they're not cared for much worse issues can develop. Size doesn't matter. Acknowledging the injury and caring for it appropriately prevents the level of severity. All of our hurts are valid no matter what measure. They are very real.
>
> **NO MORE DAD ISSUES PAGE 12**

- Describe the specific ways you were wounded in your relationship with your dad.

> "I was sitting in her office as the Assistant Principal told me I would be suspended for five days and that I was lucky not to be expelled from the school. I had really screwed up, and I knew I was going to feel so full of shame when my dad found out why and what for. I felt like a bad kid, and my dad would make me feel like a troubled individual. He could only see the wrong."
>
> **NO MORE DAD ISSUES, PAGE 78**

- How do you think your dad felt about you? Describe the attitude you carried as a result.

1 Corinthians 4:15 (MSG): *"There aren't many fathers willing to take the time and effort to help you grow up."*

- How could your dad have spent more time? How would it have made you feel?

RESOLVING ISSUES

Dave had a deficit in his heart, and he looked to his father to fill it. He expressed this in this excerpt from the book.

> "He (Dad) wasn't coming to my defense or showing any compassion for the mistreatment I'd received. The incident left me with so many questions about my dad: Don't you care? Do you love me? As a son, I felt alone and neglected.
> **NO MORE DAD ISSUES PAGE 63**

When we trust in God's love we should have no fear of loneliness, abandonment, or neglect. In this parable, Jesus is explaining how great the unconditional love of God the Father is.

> *The younger said to his father, 'Father, I want right now what's coming to me.' "So, the father divided the property between them. It wasn't long before the younger son packed his bags and left for a distant country. There, undisciplined and dissipated, he wasted everything he had. After he had gone through all his money, there was a bad famine all through that country and he began to hurt. He signed on with a citizen there who assigned him to his fields to slop the pigs. He was so hungry he would have eaten the corncobs in the pig slop, but no one would give him any. "That brought him to his senses. He said, 'All those farmhands working for my father sit down to three meals a day, and here I am starving to death. I'm going back to my father. I'll say to him, Father, I've sinned against God, I've sinned before you; I don't deserve to be called your son. Take me on as a hired hand.' He got right up and went home to his*

father. "When he was still a long way off, his father saw him. His heart pounding, he ran out, embraced him, and kissed him. The son started his speech: 'Father, I've sinned against God, I've sinned before you; I don't deserve to be called your son ever again.' "But the father wasn't listening. He was calling to the servants, 'Quick. Bring a clean set of clothes and dress him. Put the family ring on his finger and sandals on his feet. **LUKE 15:12-22 (MSG)**

- What do you treasure most in this parable?

- What do you love most about this father?

God can't love you anymore or any less. He loves you at your worst, just like he loves you at your best. Nothing will ever change that.

OVERCOMING ISSUES

King Solomon, one of David's sons who would eventually rule the Nation, shares a simple word of wisdom in this scripture: *"There is nothing new under the sun"* (Ecclesiastes 1:9)

- Does this scripture give you any type of relief in knowing you're not alone in the pain you share from your relationship with your dad? Why or why not?

- Is it possible your dad has the same hurts and frustrations as you do? What advice would you give him?

TRANSFORMING ISSUES

Our Heavenly Father promises to be our dad in ways no man on earth ever could.

"Abba" is an Aramaic word conveying a personal intimacy with a father. More than a title, he's loyal, does not harm, and will meet your every need.

- If you could get all of your heroic fatherly needs met by Abba Father, what would they be?

1 John 3:1: *"How great is the love the Father has lavished on us, that we should be called children of God!"*

- Describe what you think lavished love is like.

Write out a prayer asking God for what you need from him and what you need to be healed from.

SESSION #3

FACING HURTS FROM A FLAWED HERO (PART 2)

> "When we identify the realities of the condition in our hearts, we can find the remedies to bring healing and freedom."
>
> **NO MORE DAD ISSUES PAGE 65**

Book Reading: Part II 9-11

UNCOVERING ISSUES

Absalom grew angrier and more defiant with his dad, while Tamar was humiliated and devalued. David, the dad they wanted as a hero, just didn't do his part to address what Amnon had done to Tamar. Where was the justice? Where was the security?

The scriptures were very clear. David initially was furious when he heard of the dysfunction and crime that had happened, but then he didn't do anything about it.

How can you ever have a respectful and trustworthy relationship with a dad who doesn't show up to do his part in the home? Are you supposed to act as if nothing happened? You've been betrayed and wish the hero would've come to the rescue...but he didn't.

How are we supposed to overcome our strong emotions of wounds and frustrations from our dads? Surely, dad should fix what he did and the situation before we are required to forgive. Right?

In the pages of his book, Dave describes the common perspective most hold when it comes to forgiveness, leading us to wrestle inwardly.

> "Before we are willing to go to that place of forgiveness and reconciliation, we are certain they owe us an apology, and until then, we won't let them off the hook. All the while, we are the ones carrying pain, rehearsing pain, and praying the pain will go away. We have convinced ourselves that extending forgiveness wouldn't take the ache away. Instead, they have to be the one to admit their faults, show remorse, and ask for forgiveness. And so, we make unforgiveness our friend. As the saying goes, unforgiveness is like drinking poison and waiting for the other person to die."
>
> **NO MORE DAD ISSUES, PAGE 102**

- Do you find yourself holding these mindsets, yet you are struggling? In what ways?

- How does this wrong perspective on forgiveness, described in the excerpt, backfire and hurt us?

> We have established expectations of our dads to help us grow up. We long to be showed value, receive healthy self-esteem, gently cared for, and a sense of security.
>
> "The Apostle Paul, in his letter to the church at Ephesus, clearly pointed out where we develop rebellion and authority issues when he was admonishing the dads on how to lead. "Fathers, don't over-correct your children or make it difficult for them to obey the commandment. Bring them up with Christian teaching in Christian discipline." (Ephesians 6:4 Phillips NT).
>
> Paul said, "don't over-correct" (don't be critical, hard, harsh, controlling, etc) or "make it difficult for them to obey" (creating refusal, resentment, rebellion, strife). This is the kind of authority that crushes.
>
> Instead, he told them to use "Christian teaching" (morals, wisdom, right living), and "in Christian discipline." Discipline here, in Greek, is nouthesia, meaning put in the mind by word, or call attention to. He's encouraging dads

> to show children what to do, then reminds them to praise them to do it. This is an authority that covers."
> **NO MORE DAD ISSUES, PAGE 87**

- Do you believe your dad's way of fathering was one that "crushes" (overcorrected, made it difficult to obey)? How?

- When it comes to cooperating with authority, do you find it difficult to obey or even refuse? Describe.

- As you look over the history of your life, would you agree you've shown traces of disrespect towards authority figures (teachers, leaders, managers, etc.)? Why or why not?

> Proverbs 13:24 says, "A refusal to correct is a refusal to love; love your children by disciplining them." The word discipline comes from a Hebrew root word meaning to instruct. We want our dads to love us, correct us, and instruct us. These things bring structure and security into the homes and hearts of children. But you cannot correct what you will not confront.
>
> As we look into the behavior of David's children, we find attitudes and responses that develop as a result of a dad not "doing his job."
>
> **NO MORE DAD ISSUES, PAGE 64**

- When you read this excerpt, why does correction bring a sense of care and security?

- Do you agree with the statement, "We want our dads to…correct us and instruct us?

> "Imagine how unworthy Tamar must have felt. Absalom hated Amnon for "disgracing" Tamar, and he eventually murdered him. While Tamar likely found justice and security in her brother's outrage, I'm sure Tamar, like any child, would have preferred the intervention and presence of her dad."
>
> **NO MORE DAD ISSUES PAGE 94**

- How do you think David's absence and this assault affected Tamar's self-worth?

- Are you still hoping for the day your dad will give you the approval and worth you need? What would that look like to you?

CONFRONTING ISSUES

Honoring leaders and those in charge is such a struggle because obedience always requires trust. If you have a dad you've lost trust in or had no trust in, it almost feels impossible to trust anyone. If you've decided authority doesn't deserve to be trusted, you more than likely will not have much respect for them.

Dave mentions our dad's issues may have paved the way to troubling perspectives.

> "Are you willing to go there for a minute? Do you have signs of authority issues that may come from conflict with your dad? How are you at taking criticism? Are you ever defiant or reluctant to cooperate? Do you demand respect from others? Do you question or disregard rules? Are there any authority figures who might say you frustrate and/or upset them? Sometimes the disrespect is subtle.
>
> Many of us have issues with respect; it doesn't make you a terrible person, but how you deal with it matters. I had to look hard in the mirror to acknowledge who I really was regarding authority. You can't overcome what you won't own."
>
> **NO MORE DAD ISSUES, PAGE 86**

- Do you possess any of the issues Dave mentioned? If so, what are they, and when and where do they show up?

- Is it your tendency to take responsibility for conflicts you're a part of, whether you're in charge or not? Why?

- Are you of the belief that people who easily obey and submit to leaders are weak? Where did you get that from?

Sometimes, we feel devalued, so we are under the impression if we let someone have control, we might lose our value. It creeps in from insecurity. Unfortunately, some of these insecurities stem from our relationships with our dads.

> "When we long to feel valued by others, insecurities rush to the surface. Do you find you possess an unhealthy craving for approval? Perhaps your heart is wounded from lack of affirmation like mine was.
> Some people always have to feel "needed," and they run to the aid of others. There are others who want to be liked at any cost, so they become people pleasers.

> Others need to be the center of attention and get the credit for everything. Sometimes it's as simple as working extremely hard for the purpose of other people seeing your worth."
>
> **NO MORE DAD ISSUES, PAGE 96**

- Does your behavior with friends and acquaintances reveal you have these habits?

- How would you have felt if your dad did some of these things for you (gave affirmation, credit, attention, and likes)?

- How much stronger would you be emotionally if your dad provided a trustworthy covering that gave you approval?

RESOLVING ISSUES

> *"After his baptism, as Jesus came up out of the water, the heavens were opened and he saw the Spirit of God descending like a dove and settling on him. And a voice from heaven said, "This is my dearly loved Son, who brings me great joy." What's interesting in this scripture is Jesus hadn't started any ministry. He hadn't performed any miracles; no blind eyes had been opened, no former lame people walking, no deaf people receiving their hearing, and no one had been raised to life. Jesus was simply God's son, and he was pleased to be his father.* **MATTHEW 3:16-17 (NLT)**

- What does God the Father's words say about his heart for Jesus? Is it possible God feels the same towards you? Explain.

- Do you find it difficult to believe you bring God joy no matter what you have or have not done in your life? How do you think you developed this perspective?

- Who in your life has demonstrated they are proud of you? How did they show it?

What we learn from the heart of God is He values us just because he created us and wants to have a relationship with us.

- Is it easy or difficult to embrace this kind of heart God has for you? Why?

OVERCOMING ISSUES

Dave mentioned how he needed to forgive his dad. It was too painful to harbor the wounds and frustrations he wouldn't let go of. He was broken and needed a supernatural change to take place in his heart.

Unforgiveness is a painful load to carry. There's an old saying, "Forgiveness is setting a prisoner free and finding out the prisoner was you."

- Have you felt the pain of unforgiveness? How has it imprisoned your life?

"Get rid of all bitterness, rage and anger, brawling and slander, along with every form of malice. Be kind and compassionate to one another, forgiving each other, just as in Christ God forgave you." **EPHESIANS 4:31-32 (NIV)**

- If the negative traits listed in this passage were able to decrease due to being compassionate and forgiving, would you be willing to try? Why or why not?

TRANSFORMING ISSUES

Most people don't know this common saying came directly from the Bible in the following scripture.

Deuteronomy 32:10 (TLB) *"God protected them (children of Israel) in the howling wilderness. As though they were the <u>apple of his eye</u>."* That phrase is one explaining a person who has a sincere affinity for something or someone.

- You have value in God's eyes. He doesn't look at the bad, and he's not even looking for the bad. He sees the great promise and potential he gave you. How does that make you feel?

Forgiveness will be the greatest victory over scars and frustrations with your dad. You can't be a whole and healthy person without it.

- Are you ready to take steps to forgive your dad so you can find freedom? Why or why not?

─────── SESSION #4 ───────

SEEING THROUGH THE EYES OF MERCY

> "I don't believe forgiveness is final---but rather a daily rehearsal" **NO MORE DAD ISSUES P 109**

Book Reading: Part III (12-14)

UNCOVERING ISSUES

> The Prophet Samuel asks Jesse to a large dinner for him and his seven sons, not knowing the prophet is there to anoint the next king God has chosen. Jesse didn't even invite David to dinner with his other sons! It was as if he didn't exist. It may not sound like a huge thing, but if you were David, and you heard your dad and brothers went to a special, invitation-only dinner without you, it would injure your spirit. It wasn't as though Jesse forgot about him, either. One by one, the seven other sons passed in front of Jesse. When the Prophet asks if he has another son (kind of putting Jesse on the spot), Jesse responds by

> referring to David as "young." In the root meaning of the Hebrew word, he called him a "runt." Then Jesse mentions that David is out "tending the sheep," which was seen as a low and dirty job, a horrible, unwanted chore. Through his words and actions, it's clear that Jesse minimizes his son as if he deserves to be disqualified from the group.
>
> Jesse's obvious neglect and lack of interest begs the question, Did he not believe in his son, David? These could be general or partially true assumptions, but if you're David, this was likely a big deal.
>
> Then the exclamation point comes when Samuel rises up and anoints David to be the next king…There's no mention of Jesse celebrating, congratulating, or cheering David and his bright future.
>
> **NO MORE DAD ISSUES, PAGE 111**

- Maybe if Absalom had known about the perceived hurt David experienced, he may have been more forgiving. Are you open to gaining some understanding of any wounds your dad may have experienced? Why?

- As far as you know, what are some painful experiences your dad went through which may have contributed to the wounds you received from them?

- Have you ever reasoned your dad's past hurt is irrelevant, and you will not accept any excuses from your dad for the way he treated you? What was your justification for that view?

- Was/is your upbringing better than your dad's? In what ways?

The Bible does give a handful of helpful practices for dads to be life-giving in their role as a father. In this scripture, 1 Thessalonians 2:11-12 states, *"Like a father with his child, holding your hand, whispering encouragement, showing you step-by-step how to live well…"*

- In your opinion, what's the average score for your dad's fathering this way? Why did you give that score?

- Do you believe the directives listed in the passage are easy to accept or consider in regard to your dad? How?

CONFRONTING ISSUES

> When his mom and stepdad picked him up at Los Angeles International Airport, my dad assumed they were headed home until he noticed they were taking a different route. They weren't headed towards the Montebello area in East Los Angeles; they were venturing through the streets of downtown.

> His stepfather pulled over on 5th Street, in Skid Row—the place where transients, drug pushers, addicts, prostitutes, and drunks resided. His mother turned around to face my dad and said, "Bobby, you can't come home. He can't handle you anymore. This is where you belong." Stammering out of fear, my dad begged to come home and vowed to change. But when he realized they weren't going to budge, he climbed out of the car and entered his new home. His mom and stepdad drove off into the distance without looking back. His new life would be lived on the streets of Los Angeles, where he would fight for survival.
>
> My dad never received true caring love from a father or father figure. He only experienced abuse, neglect, and abandonment.
>
> **NO MORE DAD ISSUES, PAGES 122-123**

- If Dave's dad was just a "friend" he knew, how do you think Dave would feel once he heard this "friend's" life?

- If you have any traces of a hardened and judgmental heart, how does it affect your other relationships?

- Dave makes the statement, "When we refuse to offer mercy, we take a judgmental stand." Do you agree with him? How?

- Do you think it's possible you are being judgmental of your dad? Do you believe you have the right to take that stand? Explain.

It's easy to overlook the brokenness in someone else's life when we're so consumed with our own. It is a natural human response. But it does develop the judgmental spirit in which no one wins. Only focusing on our pain may be we carry dad issues for so long and live defeated.

An eye-opening verse gives us hope for victory. James 2:13 (NIV) says, "Mercy triumphs over judgment."

- Mercy has been simply defined as "not getting what you deserve." If you were to stop holding issues against your dad, in what ways would you possibly experience victory in your life?

- How do you think your heart would feel if you chose to have mercy on your dad?

- Do you believe your dad tried to be a good and loving dad? In what ways? How would he answer this question?

> Dr. Gary Chapman, author of the book "The 5 Love Languages" shares, "What makes one person feel loved will not make another person feel loved. We must discover and speak each other's love language." I believe my dad worked hard to love me, but he could only love me the way he craved from a father all his life. No More Dad Issues p 138 Dave also mentions, "My dad loved me from a deficit. It was a deficit I didn't comprehend or try to understand before."
> **NO MORE DAD ISSUES PAGE 127**

Dave realized his dad was incapable of loving and meeting his every need. He needed to search for glimpses of love his dad tried to give. If he chose to accept the efforts his dad did give, he wouldn't be broken by the high expectations he placed on his dad.

- Share as many ways you recall, large or small, your dad demonstrated love in his eyes.

RESOLVING ISSUES

Here's a weird question. Have you ever wondered why Swiss cheese has holes in it? Carbon dioxide given off by the bacteria used to make Swiss cheese creates air bubbles in the process. These bubbles creating "holes" are actually referred to as "eyes." It gives a totally different perspective. You focus on "holes," and you focus through "eyes."

This is a simple illustration of how we can be with our dads. We look at all the holes, hang-ups, failures, hurt, and more they've caused. We can get so focused on the holes of our dads we grow bitter or become discouraged. But if we choose to focus through the "eyes," we can see there's more to discover. Maybe if we look through the "eyes," we'll find a solid, complete, and perfect cheese on the other side. I'm referring to the Heavenly Father, who is everything our earthly dads couldn't be. Healing can't take place in your heart until you choose to fill it with God's love alone. A love that will never disappoint or go missing.

- Do you believe you have focused on the continual unresolved issues, which has only bred more frustration or bitterness towards your dad? Explain.

- Do you think you'd have more healing and freedom if you chose to look beyond your dad's ability to love and embrace God's love? How would you feel more healed and freer?

In Romans 8:38-39 (NLT), the Apostle Paul writes,

> *"And I am convinced that nothing can ever separate us from God's love. Neither death nor life, neither angels nor demons, neither our fears for today nor our worries about tomorrow—not even the powers of hell can separate us from God's love. No power in the sky above or in the earth below—indeed, nothing in all creation will ever be able to separate us from the love of God that is revealed in Christ Jesus our Lord."*

- In what ways should this unending love from God work in and through us?

The way we know God's mercy is making a difference in us is how we extend it to the world. Jesus chose mercy over judgment, even when he had the ability to judge. John 3:17 (NCV) reads, *"God did not send his Son into the world to judge the world guilty, but to save the world through him."*

- Even though Jesus refused to be on a mission to judge, why do we sometimes feel the right to judge?

- If we are to save and not judge people, in what ways does mercy "save" people?

OVERCOMING ISSUES

The incomprehensible trait about God is his ability to see the best in us even when we have committed the worst in his eyes. God has not only the strength to forgive and forget, which is humanly impossible but also his unwillingness to hold anything against us. Can you imagine if God kept a record of everything and continually brought them up whenever we failed? They would be eternally unbearable. Instead, he chooses mercy and then offers grace to discover a better life in Him.

What if breaking through dad issues included mercy for others or for your dad? What if that is what got you over the hump of dwelling on hurt, hatred, bitterness, and more? Wouldn't mercy and grace be worth it for all of us?

Philippians 2:3-4 (ESV) gives us a challenging perspective on mercy and grace.

> "Do nothing from selfish ambition or conceit, but in humility count others more significant than yourselves. Let each of you look not only to his own interests but also to the interests of others."

- How might "selfish ambition" hinder us from being merciful?

- Though it is extremely difficult at times, what do you think looking "to the interest" of your dad may be like? Why?

- Within needs to be overcome to show this type of grace and mercy?

TRANSFORMING ISSUES

Dave said his dad had loved from a deficit, trying to show love he had not known nor received.

- If we accept the fact we all have deficits of love, how would that impact the way you view your dad?

Jesus made it very clear in Luke 6:36 (AMP) what mercy includes for application but also as a gentle reminder. *"So be merciful (sympathetic, tender, responsive, and compassionate) even as your Father is [all these]."*

- Remembering how merciful God is towards you, in what ways does that motivate you to show mercy?

Breakthrough is necessary when we have a stronghold prohibiting us from implementing positive change. If you have been unable to speak or pray blessings over your dad, a breakthrough can begin in your heart right now if you practice the next exercise.

- Write out a sincere prayer of blessing over your dad.

You can do it! It is possible…because you have the great and merciful God alive and working in you!

SESSION #5

QUITTING THE BLAME GAME

> "I continued to carry the mindset he was the one that needed to change and if he did, we would live happily ever after"
>
> **NO MORE DAD ISSUES, PAGE 145**

Book Reading: Part IV (15-17)

UNCOVERING ISSUES

> The name Absalom means "Father of Peace," and yet, Absalom lived a life fueled by frustration, tension and bitterness. It's a sad reality he never experienced God-given providence over his life. Absalom could've begun a new tradition in his lineage of fathering—or perhaps started a new practice of healing, reconciliation, and restoration passed down to future generations.
>
> Instead, Absalom's life path was filled with far more conflict

> and turmoil than peace. In his eyes, his father, David, hadn't changed, so he refused to as well. It was a tragedy.
> **NO MORE DAD ISSUES, PAGE 149**

- What makes the story of Absalom's heart so sad? How could he have changed it?

- What more needs to happen before you're convinced you need change to happen, even if it means only you?

- Do you believe God has been nudging you to soften over time? What is your usual response?

Like most people, it's likely you have said in response to a past argument, "They made me mad." That's a false statement. The reality is that no one can force feelings or how they respond to you. You literally must take control of your emotions or allow them to be out of control to have your desired responses. Absalom opted to let his feelings run wild, so his actions were deadly.

If we want to override destructive feelings and behavior, we need strength beyond ourselves. This is where God's work is desperately needed. 1 John 3:20 (NLT) says, "God is greater than our feelings."

- What do you think that scripture means?

- Regarding the feelings and perspectives you have held, how do you need God's help to overcome previous patterns you repeat? What are some of the patterns?

- What do you, or have you, wrestled with when it comes to releasing your dad's offenses?

- Taking responsibility and not shifting blame is a bold decision to have victory over dad's issues moving forward. What are the differences between remaining a victim and choosing to be a victor? List some.

One of the gold standards in the hotel industry is Ritz-Carlton. For decades, they have continually evaluated their services, upgraded practices, rewarded employees, and improved the products they provide for guests. They have created a model other hotel chains look to reproduce.

There tend to be people in our lives who leave an impression on us because of the ways they control themselves and have positive outcomes.

- Who in your life has left a great impression due to how they control themselves in offensive situations? What do you admire about them in those moments?

- If you could acquire one of their attributes, which one would it be? Why?

CONFRONTING ISSUES

> It's natural for us to justify our personal opinions about situations and circumstances we face in life. We can convince ourselves we are right and everything, and everyone, should adjust. Dave had to be open to the sobering, yet relieving, approach which would bring transformation in his soul.
>
> Over time, I realized my judgment was affecting all of my relationships, and in order to move forward into health, I needed to stop focusing on the faults of others. I had a real problem with blaming others. It made me feel better temporarily but caused me to delay taking ownership of my shortcomings and prevented me from changing.

> Every time I did this, I chose to pick up past hurts and carry them into my conflicts with others. Instead of looking at what I needed to change about myself, I blamed others. I refused to realize that I was part of the problem. Had I been brutally honest, I would have seen that I was the common denominator.
>
> If I wanted my life to change for the better...it was time for me to control the controllable.
>
> **NO MORE DAD ISSUES, PAGE 157**

What good is it to be right but still have a life hampered by tension and struggles? How right are we if our reasoning continues to come with negative results? Proverbs 14:12 (NIV) states, *"Some people think they are doing right, but in the end it leads to death."* Sometimes, getting your way is still deadly in your personal life and in relationships with others.

- Are you willing to abandon what you believe is right so you have peace in your life and with others? Why or why not?

- If the hardest person to change is you, what new attitudes and actions do you need to put on?

RESOLVING ISSUES

> As I think about Absalom, I wonder how his life would have turned out had he experienced a life-changing moment like I did. His behavior had the same hardness, attitude, and resentment that mine did; he refused to let go. Perhaps, if he had received a revelation, he would have lived longer, witnessed his children growing up, found a relationship with David, and walked a path to reconciliation. Instead, he held on to the pain and bitterness that terrorized his heart.
> **NO MORE DAD ISSUES, PAGE 156**

Even if you don't have an encounter with God like Dave did, a personal decision still must be made. Simply reading this book can be that special "Ah, ha" moment for you, and work will still be necessary to move forward. You'll have to look within and see what is important for you to adjust in your heart.

"Each person should judge his own actions and not compare himself with others...Each person must be responsible for himself"
GALATIANS 6:4-5 NCV

- As we judge others, how are we comparing ourselves to them? Explain.

- If we are busy judging others, how does it impact our ability to take responsibility for ourselves?

- When it comes to conflict or hardships in relationships, are you hesitant or quick to accept responsibility for anything? Explain.

OVERCOMING ISSUES

Humble people don't make excuses; they simply are willing to see what's best in the long run and adjust where necessary. They appreciate correction, which will lead them to a more satisfying life. It requires a secure and humble person to be willing to make corrections for a brighter future. These individuals are wise.

Prideful people excuse themselves from correction and never change course. They don't like to be told what to do or where they're wrong. Proverbs 15:1 (NIV) *"He who hates correction is stupid."* Pride can be embarrassing if we choose to alter our course and perspectives.

- How do prideful people arrive at the destination of stupidity?

- What are some behaviors that reveal we are not living in humility and we're becoming prideful?

- We all have had our challenges with pride. How has pride shown up in your personal life?

> Taking on humility, which invites God's help and favor, means we come to the end of ourselves. We stop justifying our actions. We stop blaming others. We stop behaving ungodly. We stop nurturing unforgiveness.
> We admit when we've been wrong. We realize this burden is too large to bear, and we're helpless on our own. When we come to this place, God is able to repair us and prepare us for a great future of peace and grace.
> **NO MORE DAD ISSUES, PAGE 148**

- Are you willing to do what it takes to be healed from your wounds? Why or why not?

- What specific changes are necessary to move forward in freedom? List them.

The most powerful and humble person to ever walk the Earth was Jesus. He had authority over nature, created each person he met face to face, and never committed a sin. Yet he had plotted to take his life, he was betrayed, lies were manufactured about him, people tried to trap him, and He became unrecognizable due to the fierce beating he received. If anyone ever had a case to take matters into his own hands, at least one time, it was him. Yet, 1 Peter 2:23 (NLT) says, *"He did not retaliate when he was insulted, nor threaten revenge when he suffered. He left his case in the hands of God, who always judges fairly."*

- Are you convinced God will judge everyone fairly? Describe why you're convinced of that.

- Would Jesus have lost respect if he retaliated or threatened harm because of how he was treated? Why?

- Do you consider yourself weak or strong if you refuse to get revenge on others? Does it reveal pride or humility?

- How is faith demonstrated when we leave our "case in the hands of God, who always judges fairly"?

TRANSFORMING ISSUES

> In one period of my journey, to help me recover from the impact of the toxic parts of our relationship, my counselor shared a vivid illustration with me.

> As children and teenagers, we are like freshly poured, wet concrete. While concrete is wet, it is very impressionable. It receives impressions made by negative labels, harsh statements, mean treatment, and so on. She explained how there were harmful impressions made in the "concrete" of my mind and heart that affected me through the years as it dried. The only way to experience transformation was to break up the destructive concrete and replace it with fresh concrete, impressed with the thoughts God had toward me. I realized God was inviting me into a much deeper loving relationship with Him.
>
> **NO MORE DAD ISSUES, PAGE 158**

Self-talk has a powerful influence on our minds and how we see ourselves. Many times, the way we speak to ourselves would be considered verbal abuse if we were speaking to someone else the same way. It's very common for the communication, or lack of, with our dads to create these "impressions in our concrete". Romans 12:2 reads, *"Be transformed by the renewing in your mind."*

- What are some thoughts you have toward yourself that need to be removed? What are new thoughts you will replace them with?

─── SESSION #6 ───

PLANNING FREEDOM FOR A GREATER FUTURE

> "I became a servant by dismissing what I needed and wanted" **NO MORE DAD ISSUES, PAGE 175**

"A goal without a plan is only a wish" **UNKNOWN**

Book Reading: (18-19)

UNCOVERING ISSUES

You have discovered and uncovered a lot of issues in your heart as you have navigated through this study. Dave came to a sobering conclusion when it comes to moving forward for a greater future,

> Inner maturity and change continued to be a long journey. I had to undo my habit of thinking... Since God had personally given me the vision, I knew I had the responsibility to help move the relationship forward.

> My dad hadn't found what I had, so I couldn't expect him to function in our relationship according to what I envisioned.
>
> **NO MORE DAD ISSUES, PAGE 169**

- Have you ever acknowledged your willingness to face some of your issues as signs of maturity?

- How does it make you feel knowing you are maturing and becoming a better you?

- Are you willing to be the one leading the relationship you have with your father? How does this change your perspective?

- Make a list of practical ways you can make the relationship healthier and more pleasant.

Dave communicates that the way he began to lead and direct the relationship was to take on a servant's mentality. This doesn't mean you become a pushover but rather someone who will humbly do the hard work, want the best overall, and not demand anything in return.

- What does it look like to serve in a relationship with your dad?

- What's holding you back from being the leader in the relationship?

In the very beginning of the book, Dave mentions "The Big Lie" — the dad's issues go away when dad corrects them. He, in fact, learned any issues he was carrying were now his, and he had to decide what he would do to break free from them. Over time through the book, we see Dave now taking possession of the relationship for the better. Romans 12:18 states, *"If it is possible, as far as it depends on you, live at peace with everyone."*

- How do you know when you've reached peace in a relationship?

- How should you respond if the other person isn't interested in having a good and peaceful relationship?

CONFRONTING ISSUES

Dave mentions how there was a bigger picture he had to focus on, and that picture was a "make or break" decision.

> As I fully understood the larger picture and experienced freedom from the pain, I faced a dilemma. Could I accept my dad for who he was, and release the high expectations of who I thought he was supposed to be? I had these expectations my whole life. My answer was yes. Throughout my healing, I have realized God gradually moved me towards acceptance and, yes, love.
> **NO MORE DAD ISSUES, PAGE 192**

- Have you made the decision to release the expectations you have placed on your dad? How did you get there?

> Sometimes, the words go against all the earthly logic I know; the words feel almost insensitive at first because of my wounds. I recall times in my devotions when Jesus' words leaped off the pages, and I'd break down in tears. There's one passage, in Luke, where Jesus begins by saying, *"But to you who are willing to listen, I say, love your enemies!"* (Luke 6:27 NIV). After that intro, I had to ask myself the brutal question, *Am I going to listen to Jesus or listen to the wounded voices from the past?* Jesus goes on to deliver some powerful and challenging words: *"Do good to those who hate you. Bless those who curse you."* (Luke 6:28-29).
> **NO MORE DAD ISSUES, PAGE 172**

- How do you identify with Dave in this excerpt?

- Though it can be hard to listen to the strong words of Jesus, why is it important to forego your earthly logic and persevere with the words he speaks?

RESOLVING ISSUES

Dave stated in the book, "It's not God's job to change the future; it's ours."

- Do you agree or disagree with this statement? Why?

There's an interesting miracle mentioned in John 5:2-9 (NIV). A paralyzed man needs a miracle, much like those with dad issues do. He was in this state for 38 years, like many who have not resolved dad issues. Then Jesus performs supernatural work in his body like those with dad issues need work in their hearts. As you read, you'll see how the miracle is given, but it doesn't, and cannot, end there.

> *"Now there is in Jerusalem near the Sheep Gate a pool, which in Aramaic is called Bethesda and which is surrounded by five covered colonnades. Here a great number of disabled people used to lie—the blind, the lame, the paralyzed. One who was there had been an invalid for thirty-eight years. When Jesus saw him lying there and learned that he had been in this condition for a long time, he asked him, "Do you want to get well?" "Sir," the invalid replied, "I have no one to help me into the pool when the water is stirred. While I am trying to get in, someone else goes down ahead of me." Then Jesus said to him, "Get up! Pick up your mat and walk." At once the man was cured; he picked up his mat and walked."*

Notice Jesus doesn't pick him up, hand him his mat, or give him a piggy-back ride. If Jesus did, the miracle would have been useless. The man wouldn't continue to experience more and more freedom from his healing. He simply tells him, get up and go!

- What would you think about the man if he didn't get up but stayed lying down and continued begging to get in the pool even though Jesus healed him? Explain.

- How do you think this might apply to you regarding the work God has been doing and the restoration that's been taking place?

We prolong the pain and heartache if we don't take intentional steps to live whole. Healing has been taking place throughout this study. Only you decide if you will walk (live) in your healing or choose to continue dwelling and rehearsing the wounds.

- What new habits and attitudes do you need to "pick up" for you to live a future of freedom?

- During this study, have you sensed the touch of God the Father in your relationship with him? Explain.

- Have you decided to forgive your dad and now believe healing is taking place? Describe.

OVERCOMING ISSUES

> In his first book written to Timothy, the Apostle Paul is trying to teach this young leader the way to serve and gain influence with those who were older, superior, and more knowledgeable. He helped him break through this stigma lodged in his mind with the empowering words, *"Don't let anyone look down on you because you are young, but set an example for the believers in speech, in life, in love, in faith and in purity"* (1 Timothy 4:12 NIV). The vision Paul was painting for leaders was to be an example of godly conduct for others to follow, then leave the results to God.
>
> **NO MORE DAD ISSUES, PAGE 174**

- Describe different types of daily, godly conduct in action.

- What area of your life would you like to become godlier? Why?

Dave made a list of 10 practices he chose to implement to create new patterns for the future. These are important to keep you on track and avoid dysfunctional behavior in interactions with those you love. The goal is to have what the Japanese call "Kaizen," which means *continual improvement*. There's the old saying, "If you fail to plan, you can plan to fail."

- Take some time and come up with at least five practices you will implement to improve relationships. (Refer to some of the practices Dave listed on pages 182-188)

TRANSFORMING ISSUES

Colossians 1:3 describes God as, *"The Father of Compassion."* This compassion is a deep sympathy and sorrow to alleviate the suffering of another. As this Father, He is THE origin and THE source of compassion.

> This Father of Compassion…is enough to fill the unmet needs of neglect, abuse, woundedness, frustration, bitterness, resentment, unforgiveness, and pain. The striving can stop. Your search is over.
> If you give God these burdens weighing down your heart, he will bring you to a wonderful place of wholeness and freedom.
> **NO MORE DAD ISSUES, PAGE 194**

- How has this book study impacted your life?

- Have other people in your life noticed any progress? Explain.

- Imagine your life one year from now; how will your life look as a result of this experience?

IN CLOSING FROM PASTOR DAVE

I want to congratulate you and thank you.

I'm proud you have taken the bold step to find healing and freedom from issues you've had with your dad. It takes a lot of courage to confront them. As you have processed and participated in the questions, you are taking monumental steps, and shifts are taking place even though you may not see them all. I believe you will enjoy all your relationships in a healthier way. I'm so happy for you.

Thank you for traveling down this road with me. We are all together in this area. Because you and I are willing to be brave, we will lead a broken generation to freedom. We will become the models for everyone with father wounds.

So, do this one huge thing. Invite someone to be part of the movement by getting them the book "No More Dad Issues" and taking them through the study guide. You are a new and better you. You've worked hard. May God continue to bless you.

Pastor Dave

ABOUT THE AUTHOR

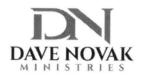

Dave Novak is a pastor, author, and speaker to this generation. His ministry has been shaped in racially diverse cultures and non-churched contexts, giving him a relevant voice of hope. In 2022, he wrote "No More Dad Issues," which focused on healing and freedom. He has been in full-time pastoral ministry for over two decades. He is the founding pastor of Streamline Church in Sacramento, CA. He and his wife Lori pastored the church for over 15 years. He is a partner to social justice initiatives globally and has served on committees for men's ministries and church plant expansion in the U.S. Dave is a nationally sought-after speaker and ordained with the Assemblies of God. Dave and Lori married in 1999 and have two young adult children, Leah and Titus.

To book Dave for events, visit Davenovakministries.com

Instagram: @TheDaveNovak

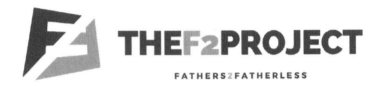

In July of 2023, Dave founded a non-profit ministry called "The F2 Project." The mission of this movement is to heal dad issues and help dads become heroes. Dave is taking this ministry into different churches, cities, and prisons with groups and courses.

To learn more about powerful ministry, visit thef2project.com

Made in the USA
Middletown, DE
30 April 2024